Happy Health For You

Olatundun Solomon

Email:olatundunsolomon@gmail.co

m

goodhealth1234567.blogspot.com

I have Honor Code Certificate from the University of Texas System edx. The course is 4.01x: Take Your Medicine-The Impact of Drug Development.

Am a Certified Alison Graduate with distinction in the course: Diploma in Nursing and Patient Care.

I have Honor Code Certificate from Harvard University through edx in the course PH201x: Health and Society.

Am a Certified Alison Graduate with distinction in the course: Diploma in Human Nutrition.

I also have Honor Code Certificate from edx Karolinska Institutet in the course KIBEHMEDx: Behavioral Medicine: A Key to Better Health.

For you to be in a position of whole physical, mental and social wellbeing is very important. Exercise makes the body physically fit. Food such as carbohydrate, protein, vitamins, fibers, minerals, fats and water keeps the mental state in proper condition. Hygiene of the environment prevents communicable diseases. Taking of bathes and washing of clothes prevents skin infections. Covering of food when it is not yet eaten prevents contamination from pathogens. Washing of fruits before eating is good habit. Cooking of meat and fish well is a method of not allowing food to be infected by pathogens (diseases causing microorganisms). Brushing of teeth with tooth brush and toothpaste prevent tooth decay. Having food recipe time table is advisable in order to eat moderately different classes of food.

Food

Food is important for the body to be healthy. The body is well nourished, the immunity of the body is high. The eyes functions well. The kidneys, liver, lungs, heart, brain and all parts of the body are in normal condition when food is eaten moderately. There are carbohydrates, protein, fats, minerals, vitamins, water and fibers.

Water is very important for the body normal functioning. It makes blood circulation to be easy. It cause hydration and prevents dehydration. It makes sweat to easily be excreted by the sweat glands, thereby regulating the temperature during hyperthermia(high temperature environment) or during exercise. Using water and soap to bath prevent skin infections. Swimming in swimming pool water, is a form of exercise. Water is used to wash fruits before eating. This prevent diseases, because the fruits are kept clean.

Carbohydrate

Energy is provided when it is eaten. These are wheat, maize, barley, yam, sweet potatoes, Irish potatoes, rice, cassava, millet and coco yam . Chiefly eaten leaving protein and other food classes in a very low state of consumption. This is an outcome of malnutrition. Eating a lot of protein such as beans, meat, fish, pea nut and other classes of food will resolve it. Over eating, especially carbohydrates can lead to obesity. Too much carbohydrate in the body turn into fat, that is stored in the body. This can lead to atherosclerosis i.e. fat accumulation in the vessels of the heart. It can also make the glucose level of the blood to be too high (hyperglycemia) which result to diabetes mellitus.

Protein

Mitosis and meiosis occurs in the body. Growth, development and repair of wornout tissues happens as a result of feeding on protein. These are egg, liver, fish, meat, and beans. Good growth is achieved when it is eaten moderately. There is poor growth when it is very little in consumption.

Fat

The human body has joints which cause locomotion of the body to happen. Fats helps in good joint movements and it aid warmth of the body. Vegetable oil is very good for the body. It prevents arthritis (inflammation of the joints) by preventing friction. It also prevents atherosclerosis(plaques in the blood vessels) because of the presence of vitamin E in the unsaturated fatty acid. This helps to prevent heart pain, that result from plaques in the blood vessels of the heart. Animal fat (saturated fatty acid) accumulate in the blood vessels after it is eaten. This makes the lumen(opening of the vessel) to be narrow(stenosis).

This results to heart pain. This can cause stroke(ischemic stroke) because of less blood supply to the brain. Stroke can result to paralysis of parts of the body. Animal fat can also cause obesity(overweight). It is preferable to go for plant vegetable oil(unsaturated fatty acid).

Fibers

Do you know that fiber is very essential for the body to prevent colon cancer? Colon is part of the large intestine of the human body. When fibers are eaten, peristalsis and segmentation occurs in the colon, which prevents colon cancer. Constipation (defecation does not occur) is prevented. Diabetes mellitus is prevented because glucose is not absorbed very high into the blood. Grounded carbohydrate food has very little fibers, this makes glucose to be easily absorbed into the blood.While chewed food such as fruits, cooked maize and yam as high fiber contents which regulates body glucose level. This is important for the body to function well.

Minerals

Electrolytes are important. Iodized salt prevent goiter (thyroid gland becomes swollen). Sea fish is good to be cooked and eaten. Eating of green vegetable helps in blood production, this prevent anemia.

Magnesium and. calcium builds bone.

Eat Food such as avocado and

bananas, they contain potassium

which is good for normal heart

function. Sodium involves in water

balance, it is found in common salt.

Phosphorus is present in bones and

teeth. Food that contain phosphorus

are fish, milk and egg. Iron functions

in blood production. Green

vegetables is source of iron.

Vitamins

The presence of vitamins in the body, result to good health. There are water soluble vitamins, which are vitamin B and vitamin C. There are also fat soluble vitamins which are vitamin A, vitamin D, vitamin E and vitamin K. Growth and development occur normally when there is sufficient amounts of vitamins in the body systems. The immunity of the body is very high, therefore the body does not fall sick.

Vitamin B prevents anemia(low blood level in the body), also it does not make beriberi to occur. Food that it can be found are green vegetables, cherry, grains, egg, fish, liver and brown rice(unpolished rice).

Vitamin C is also called ascorbic acid. It is found in citrus fruits, such as lemon, tangerine, lime and orange. It is also in guava fruit. It melts kidney stones. It prevent scurvy. Lime and honey suppress and cure fever.

Vitamin A: This aid vision. Food source are carrot, mango and pawpaw. Yellow fruits are good source of it. This makes the retina of the eye to develop normally and in good function. This prevents myopia(short sightedness) and hypermetropia(long sightedness).

Vitamin D is gotten from the sun light. Building of bone tissue occurs. Deficiency of it result to rickets and osteomalacia(soft bone formation), this can result to bow legs. Osteoporosis can also occur. This is bone becoming fragile.

Vitamin E is found in vegetable oil(unsaturated fatty acid), and also in fruits and nuts. It prevent plaques in the blood vessels. Thereby preventing hypertension(blood pressure is high than normal) that is due to narrowing of the blood vessels. It also prevents intraocular blood pressure(glaucoma).

Vitamin K prevent hemorrhage (over bleeding). When there is injury it cause clot of blood to occur. It can be gotten from green vegetables and egg.

Parts Of The Body

Organ of sight is the eyes, it is used for seeing. It has optic nerves that sends impulses to the brain.

Organ of taste is the tongue, facial nerve and glossopharyngeal nerves innervates it. The tongue is able to taste what is sweet, bitter, sour and salty.

Nose is used for smelling. Nasal receptors send impulses to the brain for interpretation.

Ear is used for earing. Impulses are sent from the ear to the brain for interpretation.

Skin is used to sense touch, temperature and pain. Motor neurons sends impulses to the brain, the brain interprets it and send it via the sensory neuron.

The liver detoxify toxins. It is involved in the digestion of food. It stores blood and glycogen(glucose that is stored in the liver).

The lungs is used for respiration. It oxygenate the blood. Oxygen is breathed into the blood and carbon iv oxide is breathed out.

The thymus and spleen functions on healthy immunity of the body. By making harmful microorganisms to be out of the body systems.

Thalamus is part of the brain, is used to regulates the body temperature.

The cerebrum is part of the brain, is used for reasoning and interpretation of informations.

The kidneys is used for filtering the blood there by preventing harmful substances from entering the blood.

The pancreas regulate the body glucose level and it functions in the digestion of food.

Cerebellum is part of the brain, is used to coordinate movement.

In male testes has sperms, this is used for reproduction.

In female ovary as ova, this is used for reproduction.

The intestines is used to absorb nutrients from the food that is eaten.

The skeleton(bone of the body) protect internal organs, gives the body shape and useful for locomotion.

The heart pumps blood to all

parts of the body.

Natural Remedies

**Temperature above 37 degree
centigrade is fever (pyrexia). Eating
of green garden egg fruits treats it.
Drinking of bitter leaf juice is also
good. I told somebody about eating
green garden egg fruits, that it treats**

fever. She ate it and the fever was treated.

Soy oil, avocado and green vegetables are good for arthritis.

Honey, bile from gall bladder of he goat and palm kennel oil resolves vermiform appendicitis. I have seen this worked effectively.

Diabetes mellitus is when the blood sugar level is more than normal. Eating of food that as normal salt, eating of cooked fish, eating of cooked beans and drinking of bitter

leaf juice can improve it.

Eating of food that as spices and

thyme is effective as anti-infective

and as antibiotic. Eating of green

garden egg, lime and honey, and

also green cucumber is good.

There was somebody having heart

pain, he ate onion and it was

resolved. Onion was used also at a

place that scorpion sting a person

and it was resolved. Food that are

good for the heart proper function

are garlic, ginger, onion and vegetables (source of vitamin E). And also fish and nuts. In addition go for exercise to keep the heart healthy.

Malaria is fever that is caused by female anopheles mosquitoes, plasmodium is sent into the blood. The therapy(treatment) for this is eating green garden egg and food that contain spices.

Under weight can be solved by eating apples, yam, rice, peanut, wheat, potatoes, beans, meat, fish, green vegetables and fruits. In addition increase water intake.

Poor eyesight can be improved by eating yellow fruits. These as beta carotene. This fruits are pawpaw, mangoes and also eating food that as the oil of red oil palm fruits.

Kidneys in the human body functions to reabsorb ions into the blood. And it excretes harmful substances from the body. When there is calculi (stones) in the kidney, it makes it not to function properly. This is called kidney stones(renoliths). Citrus fruits such as grapes, tangerines, lime, and lemon melts the stones. Drinking high content of water in this condition is good. When drug capsules are swallowed taking a lot of water is good, in order to prevent kidney stones and stone formation in the body generally.

Vitamin K stops bleeding(hemorrhage). Food that has vitamin K are banana and avocado.

Sour sop is good for cancer. Eating a lot of fruits and drinking of lots of water is good in a cancerous condition.

When there is malnutrition, eating of apple, peanut, egg, milk, soymilk, wheat and green vegetables is good.

Kwashiorkor is resolved by eating protein, such as fish, meat and beans.

High intake of fiber prevent constipation (defecation inability). Food that as fiber are whole grains, beans, legumes and fruits. This prevents constipation because it aids peristalsis and segmentation.

Goiter means struma(swelling of the thyroid gland). Putting iodized salt in food resolves this.

Electrolyte imbalance can be resolved by putting iodized salt in food, and the use of sugar in tea, eating of fruits and vegetables.

Anemia is when the blood level is below normal. Eating of cooked green vegetables as food improves it.

Also eating of green fruits is good.

This works effectively.

Colon cancer can be prevented by

eating food that has high fiber

content, such as fruits, cooked beans,

pineapple, cooked legumes and

vegetables.

When there is skin burn due to acid,

pouring a lot of water to neutralize

and pouring of egg liquid, milk and

oil is good. When there is burn

caused by hot water, pouring of egg

liquid is good.

Lack of appetite can be solved by using sugar and honey in food.

Acidosis which is acidic content of the body is high can be treated by eating cooked green vegetables helps to resolve it.

Alkalosis (alkalinity of the body is above normal) this can be resolved by eating whole grains.

Fibroid is tumor that occur at the uterus. This can be resolved by eating grape fruit.

Aloe vera is good for hair protection against infection and it is useful for hair normal growth.

Very green cucumber when sliced, is good to be rubbed on the face to prevent skin infections.

Scurvy occurs as a result of lack of vitamin C(ascorbic acid). It can be treated eating citrus fruits, such as orange, lime and lemon.

Cholera, dysentery and typhoid fever can be treated by eating food that as thyme, curry and chili. Eating lime, honey, green garden egg and very

green cucumber is very good.

Coughing(tussis) is suppressed by

eating lime, lemon and honey.

Osteoporosis makes the bone to be

fragile. This can be resolved by

eating cooked stocked fish. Boiling

of natural fresh water and allowing

it to be in room temperature.

Drinking the water, it as magnesium

and calcium which are good for

building up healthy bone. Eating of

pineapple and strawberry both as

manganese. that is good for the formation of healthy bone.

Asthma can be treated by drinking tea using the tea plant because it contains theophyline. This dilates smooth muscles. Therefore it is a bronchodilator.

Brain is an organ in the body that is very important. It interprets impulses sent to it by sensory neurons and relay it via the motor neuron. It is used for reasoning. Drinking of milk makes it very healthy. Eating honey also makes it function well.

Anemia during pregnancy can be treated by eating cooked green vegetables.

Bitter leaf(vernonia amygdalina) juice is gotten by squeezing the juice into a bowl. The juice treats anaemic dysentery, cholera, malaria fever and gut infections.

Chest pain(angina pectoris) can be treated by drinking tea made from cocoa seed, tea plant leaves and coffee seed. These contains

theobromine, this cause dilatation of

coronary artery of the heart.

Thereby resolving chest pain.

Causes Of Diseases

Unhygienic Environment: When the environment is dirty, it makes pathogens (disease causing organism) to be in such places. Thereby causing infections(communicable diseases) This can be prevented by keeping the environment clean.

Anemia: This means blood level is below normal. It can be caused by blood sucking insects, for example mosquitoes and tsetse flies. It can happened also after an injury when blood is reduced. Malnutrition also causes it. Eating of cooked green vegetables, liver and meat resolves it.

Cholera: Is caused by drinking water that contain vibrio cholerae. Boiling water before drinking, resolves it.

Kwashiorkor: This happens when there is malnutrition. There is over feeding on carbohydrates and very little feeding on protein. This results to big head appearance and big belly. It is resolved by increasing protein in the diet.

Angina Pectoris(Chest Pain): When there is accumulation of fatty plaque or blood clot in the heart vessels can cause it. Fat accumulation can be due to eating animal fat(saturated fatty acid). It is resolved by replacing animal fat with vegetable oil (unsaturated fatty acid). This as vitamin E, which prevents plaques to

occur in the vessels of the heart.

Kidney Stone: This can happen

because of undissolved drug

capsules that is swallowed. This is

resolved by drinking a lot of water.

Citrus fruits such as orange, lime and

lemon melts it. Guavas also as

vitamin C.

Goiter: This happens when there is

deficiency in iodine in the diet. There

is swelling of the thyroid gland.

Putting iodized salt in the food to be eaten solves it.

Diarrhea: This can occur by drinking dirty water. By eating food that is not well cooked, that is containing pathogens. It can also occur after infection from faeces and urine. This can be prevented by drinking clean water eating food that is well cooked. Hygiene of the body is good.

Unwashed Fruits: When fruits are not properly washed before

eating, it can result to diseases,

because they can have on them

disease causing microorganisms.

Unwashed clothes that are dirty

can harbour pathogens, that can

cause disease to the body.

Uncut finger nails that are long

can contain microorganisms that can

enter into the body when eating and

can cause infection to the body.

Over eating of refined sugar,

chocolate and carbohydrates

increase cholesterol and glucose

level(hyperglycemia). It increases body fat and it result to obesity. It can also lead to diabetes mellitus.

Cancer: Occurs when there is tumour formation. As a result of too much mitotic division of tissues. This forms new tissues that are harmful to the body. Food that as colours, additives, trans fat and various chemicals can make somebody to be at risk of cancer. Eating of soursop, apple and various fruits is good to prevent cancer. And eating natural food is very healthy.

Congenital Diseases: These are diseases that affect unborn child during pregnancy. This can occur when the mother did not eat different classes of food moderately(malnutrition). When the mother take drug, for example thalidomide can make the fetus to not have hands and legs. Drinking of alcohol during pregnancy result to fetal alcohol syndromes. Not eating enough cooked green vegetables can

result to anemia. Not eating enough

fruits can make the fetus to be

exposed to infection. Vitamins

increases the body immunity.

Food That Are Good For You.

Honey is very good to be eaten.

Too much feeding on food that as

refined sugar can cause diabetes

mellitus, hyperglycemia(high level of

glucose in the blood) and obesity(over weight).

Unpolished rice is good, it contains vitamin B which is beneficial for prevention of beriberi.

Whole grain food is good. It has a lot of fiber that prevents constipation. It also helps in the regulation of body glucose.

Food without additives is good to prevent cancer.

Fresh vegetables and fruits without preservatives is healthy.

Fresh meat without preservatives is good.

Fresh fish without preservatives is good.

Baked, boiled and steamed food not smoked is good. Smoked food can eventually lead to stroke, heart disease and lung disease.

Bread from whole grains is good.

Fruit juice with no chemical additives is good.

Vegetable oil, not animal fat.
Animal fat can lead to
atherosclerosis(fat plague in the
blood vessels) which can lead to
heart pain, hypertension and heart
failure.

Too much of egg consumption
without adding other nutritional
food can lead to increase in the
cholesterol level of the body. This
can lead to cardiopathy(heart
disease). Eat egg moderately is good
for the body.

Exercise

Moderate exercise is very good for the body fitness. The heart will function well. It prevents atherosclerosis. It prevents fatigue(weakness) in muscles, bones, cartilage, heart, kidney, liver, lungs, brain, spleen, intestine and all parts of the body.

Exercise can occur by walking distances, by jogging, stretching of the body. By pressing up. By using yo yo. And also by running.

Exercise is good for the obese, in order to reduce weight.

The lungs that are used for respiration, the heart that pumps blood to all parts of the body, the kidney that function for the reabsorption of ions into the body, the liver that functions in detoxification and for digestion and the pancreas that take part in

digestion are in good condition

when the body undergo exercise.

Taking of water during exercise is

good, because water can be out

from the body through sweat. This is

a normal mechanism to keep the

body temperature in a good state.

Fatigue is prevented through

exercise.

Sleep

Sleep is very good. It refreshes the body. It keeps the brain in good condition. It keeps the eyes and all parts of the body in good health. It makes the circadian rhythm of the body to be normal. It prevents black eyes that is due to not having enough sleep.

Your Children Health

Children needs a lot of protein for growth and development. Fish, egg, meat and beans are very good for their growth. They need exercise to keep fit. They need milk for mental health. They need all the classes of food for healthy growth.

Heredity

Gene carries hereditary information from parents to offsprings. When parents are having disease in their body system, this can be passed during pregnancy to

the child if the disease is not treated.

Prevention of diseases is good.

Cancer can be passed from parents

to child. HIV/AIDS can be passed

from parents to child. Malaria can be

passed from parents to child. Also

anemia can be passed from parents

to child.

Home Hygiene

The house is a place where the

family lives. The television, chairs,

tables, clothes, floor, wardrobes, spoons, plates, knives and shoes should be kept clean. The children's teeth should be kept clean, by brushing with toothpaste and tooth brush. This prevents tooth caries(tooth decay). Educating the children about health is good, by making them to know not to play with sharp objects that can cause infection and injury. Bathing for the children regularly prevents infections of the skin. Washing of the school bags after use is healthy.

Removing of cobwebs is healthy. Sun drying of washed clothes is healthy. Keeping sharp objects where the little children will not reach is good. Cutting of nails when long is good to prevent infections. Washing hair properly with soap and water is healthy, this prevent hair and scalp infections. Cutting of the grasses short that are in the environment around the house, prevents hiding of snakes and scorpions. This prevents snake bite and scorpion sting.

Behavioral therapy is also good.

Coming together as a family and not speaking words about sickness affecting the children in order to make them afraid. When they are afraid this can affect them psychologically. The family can go for clinical checkup in the hospital. This enable the medical doctor to diagnose and give good health informations for a healthy family. Or the family can have a family doctor to be visiting the home for regular checkups. Actions should be taken by the family, acting properly on

nutritional diets, exercises and
cleanliness in order to have a
healthy family. Parents should not
neglect their children on the aspects
of hygiene. Children should be
assisted to have proper bath, not
allowing them to injure themselves
with sharp objects that can lead to
injury and blood loss(anemia).
Planting of flowers around the house
is good. Green plants gives out
oxygen this is very good for human
use, because human breathe

in(inhalation) oxygen and breathe

out(expiration) carbon iv oxide.

Sunday	Tea, bread and egg	Rice, beans, water, fish, tomatoes and pepper	Sandwich, water and fruits

		soup.	
Monday	Dough nut, water and fruit juice	Pizza, water and soup that has fish	Potato es, water and soup having beef
Tuesday	Yam porridg e, water and	Water, whole bread and Beans	Rice, water, salad and chicke

	fruits	having thyme and curry in it.	n
Wednes day	Water, fruits, cake and tea	Water, Liver, beef, egg, pizza and green vegetab	Biscuit s, fruits and tea

		les	
Thursday	Water, Sausage, fruit juice and egg	Yam, water, vegetables, fish, tomatoes and pepper soup	Honey, water, dough nut and soup with liver in it
Friday	Milk, cocoa tea	Rice, egg, beef,	Fish, goat meat,

	and	water	turkey,
	whole	and	water,
	bread	fruits	and
			Irish
			potato
			es and
			orange
			s
Saturda y	Biscuit s, tea and fruits	Fruits, water, sandwic h, chicken	Rice, water, beans, liver with

	Breakfast	Lunch	Dinner
		and fish soup	tomatoes and pepper sauce.

The table above is recipe for breakfast, lunch and dinner. Eating food moderately as a family is healthy, by eating from all the

classes of food.

Car Hygiene

Washing the car regularly,

keeps disease causing

microorganisms out from it. This

prevents communicable diseases.

The use of sit belt during driving is good. After washing, allowing the car to sun dry is good. Disease causing organism usually use moist environment to replicate. When the car as flat tire, it should be pumped for it to be in its proper state. This prevent accident on the road. Driving car that has two side mirror makes the driver to see cars that are coming behind. The use of catalytic converter makes the smoke coming out of the car to be converted to harmless substances. Therefore preventing air pollution. Air

pollution can lead to lungs disease. It

can also lead to stroke and

suffocation.

General Health

Working for too long without resting can cause micro fracture of the bones.

Eating very late can cause stomach ulcer and intestinal ulcer. This is because the stomach secrets gastric acid.

Drinking of too much water leads to micturition(urination frequently).

Drinking of alcohol, leads to addiction and liver cirrhosis disease.

Not eating leads to hunger, dizziness, weakness and underweight.

Low level of blood(anemia) leads to body pain. And the whole body is not well nourished.

Blockage of blood supply to any part of the body leads to death(necrosis) of that part. Prevention is good by taking food that has vitamin E, e.g. vegetable oil. Drinking of cocoa tea is good it as theobromine which cause arterial dilatation.

When there is eye itching, orange is good to be eaten because it contains vitamin C.

It is good to be exposed to early morning sun because of vitamin D which is good for healthy bone formation.

During pregnancy, women should eat balance diet from the classes of food in order for the child to be born to be normal.

Regurgitation of gastric acid early in the morning that can cause chest burn can be resolved by

drinking water to neutralize it or by

drinking milk.

Eating cooked green vegetable

is good for blood formation, because

it contains folium.

During cold condition wear

Cardigan, drink hot tea and exercise

is good to keep warm.

During fever(high temperature

of the body), Eating food that as high

spice content is good.

When having black eyes due to lack of sleep. It can be treated by sleeping well.

After injury, eat more of protein because it repairs tissues. Also eat a lot of cooked vegetable soup, it leads to the production of blood from the bone marrow.

When the sugar level of the blood is too low(hypoglycemia) eat carbohydrates, honey and food that contain sugar.

Endorphins are released from the brain when you laugh and smile, this relieve pain.

Very high unhappy emotion can lead to shock. Making somebody to faint.

Taking steroids when there is no sickness for taking it, can lead to liver damage and addiction.

When somebody is in shock, cardiopulmonary resuscitation is good to be used to revive the person.

When there is excess of vitamin A, it cause loss of hair.

More than normal vitamin C consumption leads to diarrhea and dehydration.

Vitamin E in hypervitaminosis(excess vitamin) result to anticoagulant effect of blood, this makes bleeding to be excess(hemorrhage) after injury.

Calcium too low level can result to osteoporosis and cardiac arrhythmias (irregularity of the heart rhythm). When calcium is in excess it result to kidney stone (renolith) and fatigue (weakness).

Iodine in excess result to iodine toxicity (poisoning).

Environmental sanitation is good. This makes the environment to be clean. This prevent contacting disease from the environment.

During pregnancy antenatal, perinatal and postnatal care in the hospital is good.

Drinking Of enough water is good for a proper health. The blood will function well. The skin will not crack. The digestion of food will be normal. Defecation will be normal. The joints will function well. The temperature will be normal.

Brushing of the teeth with small head and with soft bristles is good. It will prevent erosion of the teeth. Using using fluoride toothpaste will prevent tooth caries.

Taking enough rest and sleeping well will make the brain to function normally and it prevent headache. This makes the circadian rhythm of the body to be kept normal. The heart will also function normal.

When parents take their bath regularly and wash their teeth in the morning after breakfast and at night after dinner it prevent disease transfer from parents to children. And when the children also bath regularly and brush their teeth in the morning after breakfast and at night

after dinner it prevent disease

transfer from children to parents.

Not eating food that has

artificial colorants, artificial

preservatives and synthetic additives

prevent cancer occurrence in parents

and children. This is because those

chemicals that can mutate the DNA

is not present in the food. This

makes the parents and children to

be healthy.

It is good not to eat too little. This prevent under weight and malnutrition. It is good not to over eat this prevent obesity, heart diseases, stroke and diabetes mellitus. When the body is obese it is good to go for exercise.

It is good to drink plenty of water after eating. This helps to prevent calculi(stone) formation in the body. Calculi can make blood vessels to be narrow and it can lead to high blood pressure(hypertension). This can lead to angina pectoris(heart pain). If not treated it can result to heart failure. This can lead to necrosis of the brain(brain death). Calculi can also form in the kidney. When this occurs it lead to urine incontinence. This means urine will not be able to be passed out. It is good to drink enough water for these to be prevented.

It is good to wash the hands frequently, this prevent disease transfer from person to person through hand touch.

Parents should remove the diaper of baby after it is dirty. And wash the buttocks and anus with mild soap and water. This prevent infection of the baby by pathogens (disease causing microorganisms). This also prevent disease transfer from child to the mother.

It is good not to smoke cigarette. This prevent cancer of the lungs. It also prevent stroke. It also prevent

liver and blood diseases.

It is good to brush the teeth

well using mirror to look at the teeth

to see that there is no particles of

food in it. This prevent acid

formation in the teeth that can lead

to demineralized teeth, tooth decay

and tooth capitation.

It is good to eat a lot of fruits

and vegetables. This makes the

immunity of the body to be high.

This makes the body to fight against

infections, thereby making the body healthy. The body can function normally.

It is also good to go to the hospital to see the medical doctor for checkup. This makes the medical doctor to diagnose and assist in making sure the body is healthy.

It is good to eat fruit and vegetable salad. This makes the body to have a lot of vitamins and minerals that will make the bones to be strong and the muscles to be healthy. This makes the body to be healthy. Fish makes the bones to be strong. Cucumber and lettuce has calcium and magnesium that makes the bone to be strong.

Egg has vitamin A(egg yolk). This makes the eye to function normally. And the growth of the body will be normal. Egg is good for the children for good growth and development. Fish and beans is also good for the children to grow normally. Exercise is good for the children. It makes them not to be overweight(obese). It makes them to be free from heart diseases. Milk is also very good for the children for a healthy growth. Soy milk and soy oil is very good it prevent heart diseases.

Too much sugar in food can result to diabetes mellitus and obesity. It can lead to disease of the retina which can result to poor sight. It is good to use brown sugar moderately. It is good not to use synthetic sweeteners. This prevent

cancerous cell formation in the body.

It is good not to allow sharp

objects to be in the floor in the

house. It can cause trauma(injury) to

the children in the house.

It is good to guide the children

when brushing the teeth. Makes

them not to injure their gums. This

also prevent teeth erosion. This

prevent bleeding gums. And it makes

the children to brush their teeth well.

This prevent mouth infections. And

it also prevent metastasis of infection from the mouth to other part of the body.

It is good not to eat very late. The stomach has gastric acid which can cause stomach ulcer. It is good to eat early and drink enough water so as to prevent stomach ulcer. Eating early also prevent regurgitation of the gastric acid from the stomach into the esophagus, which can lead to heart burn and changing of the structure of the esophagus. Ulcer of the esophagus is prevented. Intestinal ulcer is prevented.

Tea and cocoa is very good to prevent heart pain. The presence of theobromine makes cocoa and tea prevent heart pain. Eat enough cooked fish also helps to prevent heart pain because of the presence unsaturated fatty acid which helps to prevent atherosclerosis(fat accumulation in the blood vessels) this present narrowing of the blood vessels. Hypertension is then prevented. Heart pain is prevented. It is also good to drink enough water to prevent heart pain. Exercise is also good to prevent heart pain. The vessels of the body will be normal. There will be no stenosis of the blood vessels(narrowing of the blood vessels). This makes the heart to function normally. Heart diseases is prevented. Also brain diseases is prevented.

It is good for you to have your own hair clipper for your hair cut. This prevent pathogens. Pathogens will not be transferred from dirty clippers to the head. It is good to clean clippers, in order to prevent infections from dirty clippers. After using the clippers it is good to wash the hair with soap and clean water. This makes the head to be clean. It is also good to wash the neck with soap and clean water.

It is good to use vegetable oil and use fish and vegetables to make soup this makes the skin to be healthy. It prevent skin breakage. It is good to have good exercise, rest well and sleep well this makes the body to have a healthy skin. It is good to rub sliced very green cucumber on the skin of the face to clear off skin diseases. Also aloe vera is very good to treat skin infections. Also drink enough water the skin will be healthy and beautiful.

Don't chew ice it can cause teeth breakage. Don't use sharp objects on the teeth it can cause injury(trauma). When there is injury, there can be blood loss which can lead to anemia(low blood level in the body). This can result to pain in different parts of the body. This can make the body to be weak and unhealthy.

Don't over use salt in food, it can lead to hypertension. It can also lead to vomiting.

Don't use tetracycline when the medical doctor did not prescribe it to you. It can result to teeth discoloration.

After eating sweet food, it is good to gargle the mouth with clean water and swallow it. It is also good to brush the teeth with fluoride toothpaste and tooth brush. Gargle the mouth with clean water and spit it out. This prevent acid formation in the mouth which can lead to dental cavity.

It is good to go regularly to the hospital for regularly mouth cleaning. This makes food particles not to be present in the mouth. This prevent mouth infections and diseases.

It is very good to use clean water to wash the clothes. To bath, to cook and to wash the house. This prevent infections in the house.

It is very good to eat natural food. Drink enough water. Avoid eating and drinking synthetics. It makes you very healthy and your

immunity will be high.